Essential Oils for Survival

How To Assemble Alternative Remedies For A Perfect Bugout Bag

by Ann Sullivan

Published in USA by:

Ann Sullivan
217 N. Seacrest Blvd #9
Boynton Beach
FL 33425

© Copyright 2016

ISBN-13: 978-1539971665
ISBN-10: 153997166X

Table of Contents

Introduction

What are essential oils and why would they be essential in a survival situation?

When it comes to a major natural or man-made disaster, pharmaceutical supplies will likely be limited or eliminated altogether; essential oils, along with other alternative medicines, will be essential to survival. When medical access is obsolete, alternatives to our modern-day standard will keep you and your loved 1s happy and healthy.

These oils are deemed "essential," because the oils are composed of the "essence" of the plant. The difference between essential oils and other oils – like olive oil or vegetable oil, for instance – is that essential oils have high volatility and reduced fixation, which results in faster evaporation, enabling their popular use in aromatherapy. Even at high temperatures olive and vegetable oils do not evaporate.

Essential oils can be used as a supplement and as an alternative in the medical kit. Before dismissing essential oils, do a little research into the average century-old medical text; essential oils, herbs, and plenty of other natural ingredients have been used for thousands of years to treat any number of ailments and injuries. Though this sort of medicine is considered "alternative" now, it was once the gold standard. Perhaps it still should be, as these natural age-tested remedies can treat, or help treat everything from headaches to cuts and bruises to serious diseases.

Most people do not realize that they already use essential oils every day. They are in perfumes, shampoos, soaps, ointments...they are even used in furniture polish. Why are they used in so many aromatic products? Because essential oils are super concentrated aromatic liquids, so their scent is ultra-potent. Let's put this into perspective: to steam tea, use a few leaves of peppermint or juniper; to produce a single ounce of essential oil, 5 whole *pounds* of peppermint or juniper leaves are used. Some sources claim that to produce twelve pounds of essential oil would require an acre of peppermint, juniper, or any other essential oil being mass produced. These concentrated versions of essential oil are not often sold in bulk; instead essential oil is often sold in easily carried small, dark bottles, perfect for the average GOOD bag (Get Out Of Dodge). That is exactly what this book is aiming to help with; assembling an essential oil survival kit.

In the *Essential Oils Survival Kit*, we will be taking an in-depth look at essential oils and their wellness applications. First, we will discuss from where essential oils originate, how they are extracted, and the different methods of administration. Next, we will look at the various benefits of essential oils and their properties. We will then discuss the base components of "mainstay" oils; these are the basic essential oils that readers will want to consider storing in their survival kit. Lastly, we will provide a number of recipes and wellness treatments, both for pure oils and blends.

Chapter 1:
The Ins & Outs of Essential Oils

Where do essential oils come from?

Plants and plant species naturally produce essential oils for various reasons, 1 being to draw pollinator insects to them, another being to repel invading organisms (bacteria, animals). A number of chemical compounds compose each plant's essential oil, the combination of these compounds being specific to each oil. Essential oils can be harnessed from all sorts of plant components, including flowers, leaves, bark, fruit, roots, and resin. For instance, cinnamon oil is extracted from bark, lemon oil from the peel, and lavender oil from flowers. Certain plants can produce a variety of different essential oils, which are acquired from different parts of the plant. Some of these parts produce a large amount of oil, while others produce just a smidgen. The oil's quality and potency depends upon a number of factors, including the sub-species of the plant, its soil conditions, the time of year, and even the time of day it is harvested.

How are essential oils extracted?

Essential oils can be extracted from their plants by a variety of methods, including pressing, distillation, solvent and maceration. Let's take a brief look at these methods:

Pressing Method

Commonly used with citrus fruit, the pressing method extracts the oil through a technique involving pushing the fruit peels through a press. Oily fruits and plants are best suited for this technique. Orange oil for example, is extracted from orange peels, through the pressing method.

Distillation Method

This technique harkens back to the days of moonshiners, as the same sort of method used to create strong liquor can be used to extract essential oils. Using a still, boiled water and plant materials will create steam, which is then cooled by coils and condensed into a combination of water and oil. This combination does not mix, so the oil can then be extracted from it.

Solvent Method

Through a multi-step process, certain plant and flower oils can be extracted using alcohol and other solvents, which extort the essential oil from the plant materials.

Maceration Method

When a "carrier," fixed oil, or lard is mixed with the plant material and set out in the sun, over a period of time, the carrier oil is infused with the plant's essence. Heat sources, other than the sun, are often used to speed the process. Throughout the process more plant material is added to produce a more potent oil.

How do you use essential oils?

Although some studies about the effectiveness of essential oils are conducted by small companies, or even individuals, a number of them are conducted by the food and cosmetic industries. In general, the pharmaceutical industry shows next to no interest in herbal medicine, primarily because there are few options to patent such products. As such, the product's lack of profitability results in a lack of research funding. Regardless, the historical use of essential oils tells us much of what we need to know; they work and have for centuries. The qualifications of essential oils can be plotted in the survival of the human race across cultures and generations.

Another reason that studies on essential oils have not resulted in much conclusive evidence of their overall effectiveness is because definitive results are sometimes difficult to prove, as each batch of oil's qualities vary for a number of reasons. 1 is that essential oils are impossible to standardize. As menti1d above, even the slightest variance in soil conditions and the time of harvesting, as well as innumerable other factors, will produce a different product quality and potency. In addition, essential oils are often obtained from various species of the same plant; Eucalyptus Radiata and Eucalyptus Globulus, can both be used in Eucalyptus oil and as a result, they may have slightly different properties and degrees of effectiveness.

Just as there are a number of methods by which to extract essential oils, there are a number of methods to administrate them therapeutically. The variety of chemical compounds in each essential oil means that their benefits and application also vary across the board. Below are a few of these methods.

Topical Administration

Direct application of essential oils works incredibly well, as skin absorbs chemicals and other things (sunlight, for instance) like a sponge. Topical application is best for clearing up an ailment on the skin, or in the underlying muscle tissue. When applying topically, either massage the oil into the skin, or simply place on the skin for therapeutic results. Combine the essential oil with a carrier oil for topical use in order to dilute potency. This is safer, as the oil is concentrated. Rashes or muscles may be treated in this manner; always test the patient for allergens before applying. Adverse effects are produced by natural chemicals as much as synthetic 1s; poison ivy, for example.

To test for allergens, place a drop or 2 on the patient's inner forearm. If a rash develops within 12 to 24 hours, then the patient is allergic. In addition, phototoxicity – sun exposure resulting in an exacerbated burn – may be an issue when citrus oils are applied topically. 1 must proceed with caution when applying essential oils using this method.

Inhalation Therapy

Commonly known as "aromatherapy," this essential oil treatment is effective for inner ailments, like sore throat or cold. In a steaming bowl of distilled, or sterilized water, add a few drops of essential oil and with a towel over your head, bend over the bowl and inhale. The towel captures the vapors, making the technique even more effective. Essential oils can also be placed in a diffuser, or potpourri, throughout a room to produce somewhat diluted therapeutic effects.

Ingestion

When using this method proceed with caution. Direct ingestion of essential oils must be monitored and used in small doses that are diluted in a tablespoon or more of a carrier oil, like olive oil. If unsure of dosage amounts, make a tea with the relevant herb instead. Although the effects of this dilution may be weaker, this treatment is a better alternative than an overdose of essential oils.

Chapter 2:
Benefits of Essential Oils

We would not be recommending the use of essential oils if they were not beneficial to overall wellness; but in what way(s) they *are* beneficial.

Injuries and Bites

First of all, they are essential to healing injuries when pharmaceuticals run dry in a survival situation, or simply when an injury needs treatment. For instance, lavender oil is often used to prevent swelling, pain, wound infection, bleeding, scarring, and to heal wounds quickly. Essential oils are particularly helpful when it comes to disaster scenarios, offering relief from the stress, bites from insects, or animals while in the isolated wilderness. Peppermint oil will stave off migraines with just 1 or 2 drops applied topically, leaving the patient clear-headed to think strategically and lead the group, or themselves, to safety; and the same oil can also be used to remove ticks.

These are just a few oils and their uses. These same oils can serve dozens of additional purposes and help heal further injuries. The applications of other various oils are endless.

Infectious Disease

Frankincense and lemon oils can be used to reduce or eliminate cold and flu symptoms. They can also be used with any other bacterial, viral, or fungal infection. These essential oils can be applied topically over the glands, throat, feet or other areas of infection; they can also be taken internally with tea or homemade capsules. Digestive issues, such as vomiting, nausea, or diarrhea can also be treated with peppermint oil, rubbed on the belly or feet. Respiratory congestion is served well by frankincense, while sinus congestion can also be treated with peppermint oil. We will discuss the specific details of various oils and their applications in the following chapter.

Replacement for Prescription Drugs

1 practical benefit of using essential oils is their substitutive nature; they can replace Rx drugs, which is the ultimate reason to understand their application and to begin stockpiling an essential oil supply. 1 of the potential threats of economic, or social collapse, is the lack of resources; primarily the inability to procure prescription drugs. As such, finding suitable alternatives should be a priority when prepping for the worst.

Their portability is also a major bonus when it comes to survival prepping. The fact that these ultra-concentrated oils take up little-to-no space makes toting them to a survival shelter all the simpler should the need arise. The application used in most essential oil treatments requires only a drop or 2 of oil, which means that a tiny bottle will be long-lasting.

Cheap, but Effective Alternative

Though m1y may be the last thing thought of when it comes to prepping for a survival situation (m1y may even be obsolete when living through social collapse), it is worth noting that the expense of essential oils pales in comparison to prescription drugs. In fact, whether or not a person is forced to survive on essential oils due to lack of prescription reserves, they might consider substituting prescriptions for these inexpensive alternatives. Essential oils are a cost efficient, yet equally effective alternative to prescription medicine.

No Expiration Date

Another benefit of essential oils is that they do not expire, nor do they have "proper storage" requirements. A number of medicines, and medicinal products, must be replaced every couple years; this sets essential oils ahead of the pack when it comes to shelf life.

Versatility

Essential oils also have great versatility. Apart from therapeutic uses, essential oils can be repurposed for household and hygienic uses. For instance, for dental hygiene, clove oil is your go-to essential oil. To maintain skin health, frankincense and lavender will do the trick; the latter also serves as sunscreen, so it can prevent sun damage as well.

When it comes to the house or shelter, use essential oils to deodorize a number of things, which will come in handy in a disaster scenario when things start to smell bad due to lack of proper utilities and care. For example, after the 2011 tsunami and the subsequent nuclear reactor meltdown in Japan, a nurse named Risa Nakahira used essential oils to deodorize and sanitize putrid public bathrooms in overpopulated evacuation facilities. As relief workers searched for survivors, often wading through debris and decaying, Nakahira also deodorized their boots and masks using these go-to essential oils. The possibilities of these natural oils are endless.

They are also versatile when it comes to the range of patients they are capable of serving. Every1 from a great grandfather to an infant baby can be treated with essential oils in the appropriate dosage. They even come in handy when treating livestock or pets. From teething infants to dementia in the elderly, from teenagers with acne to dogs with urinary tract infections, essential oils can serve any patient with nearly any ailment.

Chapter 3:
Mainstay Essential Oils & Their Applications

Several essential oils should be mainstays in a survival kit, as they are widely versatile when it comes to their therapeutic application. Their base properties serve a number of purposes. Below we have listed these mainstays and their common uses.

Lavender Oil

Even those who are not very well-versed in essential oils know that lavender oil is significantly useful.

Lavender's natural calming effect makes it a common ingredient in herbal teas that, when drank, will help relieve stress, depression, and insomnia. Lavender oil can also be inhaled for decongestion and can be effective to cure Athlete's foot or similar rashes. This versatile oil also treats pain, stimulates the immune system, and can be used as an antiseptic, in addition to its skin care uses that help heal burns, scrapes, bruises, acne, bug bites, and rashes.

Peppermint Oil

A number of the therapeutic benefits of peppermint oil have already been menti1d in this book; however, further applications include everything from antibacterial, antiseptic, decongestion, and anti-emetic uses. When directly applied to the stomach, peppermint oil can placate irritable bowel syndrome, abdominal cramping, heartburn, and other digestive disorders. Sometimes used for headaches or migraines, simply massage a couple drops into the temple of the patient. Achy muscles, abdominal issues, painful joints – all can be treated through topical application on the affected area. As an anti-emetic, peppermint oil will help cease vomiting.

Eucalyptus Oil

Whereas lavender has a calming effect, eucalyptus has a cooling effect on the skin. Eucalyptus oil can be used as a decongestant, an antiviral, and an antiseptic.

Colds, flus, sore throats, bronchitis, coughs, sinusitis, and hay fever can all be prevented and treated with Eucalyptus. Use it to boost the immune system or treat respiratory issues. Often added to baths and used for steam inhalation and massages, the versatility of eucalyptus makes it a mainstay in any survival kit. This oil particularly benefits throat problems, and a diluted form is even used in cough medicines. Do not ingest in its pure form.

Lemon Oil

Household cleaners are no stranger to this essential oil. Lemon oil has been used for decades in household products and furniture cleaners as a surface disinfectant. Like lavender oil, lemon oil is said to have a calming effect, which is 1 reason why some companies use it to clean, or scent their offices; it provokes a calm environment, thereby improving demeanor in employees, which makes for better results in the employees' work. This oil is phototoxic: do not apply topically to the skin if under direct sunlight for an extended period of time.

Melaleuca (Tea Tree) Oil

Often found in a diluted form, combined with carrier oils (particularly fractionated coconut oil). Tea Tree oil is especially effective with skin issues, like bites, acne, skin wounds and athlete's foot. Respiratory congestion can be treated by Tea Tree oil through inhalation therapy, while topical use against fungal infections and Staphylococcus have been proven effective. Tea Tree oil can even treat femi9 issues, such as yeast infections; a vaginal douche can be produced from a few drops diluted in a pint of water. This organic oil can further be used in the garden to control pests. Proceed with caution when ingesting, or topically applying high concentrations of Tea Tree oil around sensitive areas (the eyes, for instance), as it can be toxic.

Chamomile Oil

The calming effect of chamomile is evident while drinking just a single cup of chamomile tea. This oil can be especially useful when treating children through aromatherapy. 2 main versions of chamomile oil exist: German and Roman. German Chamomile can be a bit harsh; while Roman oil is often watery. Skin conditions, like allergic irritations and eczema, can be treated effectively by chamomile, while gastrointestinal irritation and inflammation can be reduced significantly by the use of this oil.

Clove Oil

The most significant uses of clove oil are antimicrobial and as an anesthetic. Clove oil is a multi-purpose oil with uses as a sedative, anti-fungal, antiviral, antiseptic, and analgesic. The oil's natural pain relief properties make it especially useful for dentists the world over, and it can further be used in dental health by combining the oil with baking soda; the zinc oxide powder and the oil combine to create an effective temporary cement for loose crowns and lost fillings. As with many essential oils you should proceed with caution when using, as too much may irritate the gums.

Rosemary Oil

This multi-use oil serves as an anti-fungal, antibacterial, anti-parasitic and disinfectant. A few drops diluted in water produces a convenient and capable mouthwash. Constricted respiration and congestion can be relieved through inhalation. Rosemary oil, diluted with carrier oil, can also treat muscle aches or migraines, and has the capacity to get rid of spider mites in gardens.

Geranium Oil

If infected with head lice, a few drops of geranium oil in an average portion-size of shampoo can be used to treat the condition. Also use when bruised or bleeding, as geranium oil may have hemostatic properties (blood-clotting). Though the effectiveness varies between geranium species, geranium oil impedes sebum in the skin, which is useful in controlling acne issues.

Arnica Oil

This topical treatment for muscle aches and injuries serves as an anti-inflammatory and analgesic, and is used in many sport's ointments. The treatment is effective, but not long-lasting, and requires frequent application for long-term relief. Caution: do not use in aromatherapy – Arnica oil is toxic when inhaled.

Oregano Oil

Oregano oil can be used as an antiseptic and an antibacterial agent. Derived not from the oregano plant used in cooking, but from a separate species of plant, this oil is still safe to ingest; in fact, has digestive properties, as it has been found to relieve sore throats and upset stomachs. When used diluted with carrier oil, or used topically as an antibacterial, it can relieve skin infections. If applying oregano oil regularly, supplement the application with iron, as oregano limits the body's ability to absorb iron.

Helichrysum Oil

1 of the strongest anti-inflammatories and analgesics on the list, helichrysum oil can be used in massage therapy to help treat tendonitis, arthritis, fibromyalgia, and carpal tunnel syndrome. The topical properties may also keep chronic skin irritation in check.

Frankincense Oil

With uses beginning all the way back in ancient Egypt, the documented application of frankincense oil has a 5000-year history. Frankincense has been known to relieve stress, anxiety, and depression. When topically applied, the antifungal and antibacterial properties treat wounds, and when used as an inhalant, frankincense aids nasal and lung congestion.

Clary Sage Oil

The chemical composition of clary sage is very similar to estrogen and can be used to impact menstrual irregularities, hormonal issues, and premenstrual syndrome (PMS). The sedative effect of clary sage can further its use as a calming agent, and the mild effectiveness as an anticoagulant makes it a decent substitute as a blood thinner.

Thyme Oil

When it comes to thyme oil, this natural antimicrobial is almost unparalleled. Thyme can treat ringworm, athlete's foot, and other skin infections, as well as upper respiratory infections and congestion when used in inhalation therapy. Thyme is also valuable in massage therapy and can relieve intestinal cramps.

Neem Oil

The Neem tree, common in its native India, is known as "the village pharmacy" for its incredible number of chemical ingredients. More than 150 chemical ingredients are produced by this tree, and most Ayurvedic alternative remedies are largely composed of some form of Neem oil. The wellness benefits are innumerable and include treatment for just about every ailment and every organ system. Used as an organic pesticide, it can eliminate pests in a vegetable garden with a few drops of Neem Oil diluted in water. When ingested, however, this oil may be toxic.

Blue Tansy Oil

Blue Tansy is another natural pesticide, which is often planted as a "companion plant" for pest control in the garden. Used for decades to treat intestinal worms, Blue Tansy can help treat many parasites, and has also been used as an antibacterial in dental procedures. Camphor – an offshoot of Blue Tansy – can be found in ointments and chest rubs.

Wintergreen Oil

This proven analgesic and anticoagulant is composed of natural salicylates. A single fluid ounce of Wintergreen Oil equates the potency of 171 aspirin tablets. Therefore, only ingest this oil in tiny amounts. Wintergreen oil may also be effective when it comes to reducing blood pressure in hypertensives, as well as relieving intestinal spasms.

Things to consider...

Oftentimes essential oils are manufactured as blends of several pure oils. The downside to these "blends" is that the more oils added to the mix, the higher the probability that a patient may react negatively to the blend. There is also the possibility of phototoxicity.

There are also some adverse effects to using pure essential oils. They should not be used when pregnant. Allergic reactions may occur, especially when applied topically. Always use the allergy test previously menti1d before committing fully to topical treatment. When used with other medications, essential oils may react negatively. If on any current prescription medications, or have a chronic illness such as high blood pressure, epilepsy, or liver disease, then researching the effects of essential oils against personal medical history is essential to proper usage.

Regardless of these possible effects, essential oils are a viable option for treating a number of conditions. Those looking to treat, or maintain their own personal health, or that of their families, should become educated on the uses of essential oils, their natural remedies, and the methods of treatment. Only then can they begin building an essential oil survival kit.*Prior to each meal, apply 1-2 drops to your drinking water.*

Chapter 4:
Recipes for Essential Oils

As we have discussed, there are many uses for pure essential oils. Additionally, "blends" – or combinations of various essential oils – provide for further treatments of various maladies. In this chapter, we will discuss several pure essential oil uses for various medical issues, after which, we will provide a number of recipes for DIY blends that can be mixed together with the mainstays in an essential oil survival kit.

Pure Essential Oil Treatments

Arthritis

Essential oils suggested to treat this medical condition:

Lavender, German Chamomile, Rosemary, Eucalyptus, Juniper

Suggested methods of application:

Massage, Bathing, Compress

Helpful hints:

In 10 mls. of Lavender Body Oil, put 5 drops of German Chamomile in Jojoba and rub into affected area.

Back Pain

Essential oils suggested to treat this medical condition:

Lavender, Roman Chamomile, Rosemary, Marjoram

Suggested methods of application:

Massage, Bathing, Compress

Helpful hints:

For pain relief, rub 1 capful of Pain Relief Blend Oil into affected area.

Bites & Stings

Essential oils suggested to treat this medical condition:

Lavender, Peppermint, Eucalyptus, Peppermint, Lemongrass, Tea Tree

Suggested methods of application:

Massage, Compress, Direct Topical Method, Spritz

Helpful hints:

On a cotton ball or q-tip, place 1 drop of Lavender and apply to the affected area.

Bruises

Essential oils suggested to treat this medical condition:

Lavender, Roman Chamomile, Juniper, Lemongrass

Suggested methods of application:

Massage, Cold Compress

Helpful hints:

Place 1 drop of Roman Chamomile into Jojoba and rub over affected area.

Cold Sores

Essential oils suggested to treat this medical condition:

Eucalyptus, Patchouli, Geranium, Bergamot, Sandalwood

Suggested methods of application:

Direct Topical Method

Helpful hints:

On a cotton ball or q-tip, place 1 drop of Geranium and apply to the affected area.

Common Cold

Essential oils suggested to treat this medical condition:

Lavender, Lemon, Eucalyptus, Cedarwood

Suggested methods of application:

Massage, Inhalation, Vaporization, Tissue

Helpful hints:

To relieve cold symptoms, vaporize 6-8 drops of a Respiratory Blend solution.

Dermatitis

Essential oils suggested to treat this medical condition:

Lavender, Roman Chamomile, German Chamomile, Patchouli, Sandalwood

Suggested methods of application:

Massage, Bathing, Exfoliate, Compress

Helpful hints:

For pain relief, add to Jojoba and rub into the affected area.

Fluid Retention

Essential oils suggested to treat this medical condition:

Frankincense, Juniper, Grapefruit

Suggested methods of application:

Massage, Bathing, Foot Bath, Compress,

Helpful hints:

In the shower, exfoliate your entire body with Detox Body Polish.

Hay Fever

Essential oils suggested to treat this medical condition:

Eucalyptus, Roman Chamomile, German Chamomile, Lavender

Suggested methods of application:

Tissue, Inhalation, Vaporization

Helpful hints:

For temporary relief of a runny nose, place 1 drop of Peppermint onto a tissue and inhale.

Headache

Essential oils suggested to treat this medical condition:

Peppermint, Basil, Orange, Lavender, Bergamot

Suggested methods of application:

Massage, Inhalation, Vaporization, Tissue

Helpful hints:

For pain relief, add 2 drops of Peppermint to 10mls of Lavender Body Oil, and apply to temples while avoiding the eye area.

Head Lice

Essential oils suggested to treat this medical condition:

Lime, Tea Tree, Eucalyptus, Lemon,

Suggested methods of application:

Hot Oil Treatment, Hair Rinse, Spritz

Helpful hints:

For prevention of head lice, dilute 6 drops of oil into 100 mls. of water and spritz the scalp daily.

Indigestion

Essential oils suggested to treat this medical condition:

Lime, Mandarin, Lemongrass

Suggested methods of application:

Massage, Compress, Vaporization, Tissue

Helpful hints:

To relieve indigestion, rub 1 drop of Mandarin in Jojoba over the affected area.

Insomnia

Essential oils suggested to treat this medical condition:

Orange, Lavender, Mandarin, Neroli, Marjoram,

Suggested methods of application:

Vaporization, Bathing, Tissue

Helpful hints:

Just before you lay down to sleep, dispense a single drop of Lavender onto a tissue and place inside the top of your pillow sheet.

Menopausal Symptoms

Essential oils suggested to treat this medical condition:

Lavender, Russian Chamomile, Clary Sage, Geranium, Jasmine

Suggested methods of application:

Massage, Bathing, Vaporization, Compress, Spritz

Helpful hints:

To relieve hot flashes, combine Lavender and Peppermint in a spray bottle to create a spritz.

Muscle Soreness

Essential oils suggested to treat this medical condition:

Lemon, Eucalyptus, Grapefruit, Lemongrass, Rosemary

Suggested methods of application:

Massage, Bathing, Compress

Helpful hints:

To prevent muscle soreness and straining, apply Muscle Easy Body Oil to the affected areas before exercise.

PMS

Essential oils suggested to treat this medical condition:

Clary Sage, Geranium, Neroli, Lavender, Rose

Suggested methods of application:

Massage, Bathing, Compress, Vaporization

Helpful hints:

Over the heart, rub 1 drop of Rose in Jojoba to improve balance.

Scars

Essential oils suggested to treat this medical condition:

Lavender, Frankincense, Sandalwood, Patchouli

Suggested methods of application:

Massage, Direct Topical Method

Helpful hints:

On a cotton ball or q-tip, place 1 drop of Lavender onto cotton bud and rub into affected area.

Sinusitis

Essential oils suggested to treat this medical condition:

Tea Tree, Eucalyptus, Peppermint

Suggested methods of application:

Tissue, Inhalation, Vaporization

Helpful hints:

For temporary relief, place 1 drop of Peppermint onto tissue and breath, avoiding skin contact.

Stress

Essential oils suggested to treat this medical condition:

Bergamot, Lavender, Sandalwood, Neroli

Suggested methods of application:

Massage, Bathing, Vaporization, Inhalation

Helpful hints:

To relieve stress, dispense 1 drop of Bergamot onto a tissue and inhale regularly.

Sunburn

Essential oils suggested to treat this medical condition:

Peppermint, Lavender, Roman Chamomile, German Chamomile, Tea Tree

Suggested methods of application:

Cold Compress, Bathing

Helpful hints:

Dilute 6 drops of Lavender with water in a spray bottle and regularly spritz atop affected area.

Blended Oil Treatments

Insomnia Blend

Ingredients

4 ounces vegetable oil

15 drops bergamot oil

10 drops sandalwood oil

10 drops lavender oil

3 drops frankincense (optional)

2 drops ylang ylang oil

Directions

Whether for chronic insomnia, or simply having trouble falling asleep, you can sleep easy with this Insomnia Blend. Mix all ingredients together and use either topically as a massage oil, or in the bath. 2 teaspoons in bathwater will suffice. To personalize the blend, add 2 additional drops of whatever oil is desired; for instance, rose or jasmine will give the blend a pleasant scent.

Remove the vegetable oil from this recipe, and it can be used in a potpourri cooker, or aromatherapy diffuser, or simply simmer the blend in a pan of water for aromatic effect.

Nausea Aromatic Blend

Ingredients

2 drops vegetable oil

2 drops lemongrass oil

2 drops chamomile oil

1 drop fennel oil

Directions

The nausea aromatic blend serves nausea, appetite loss, gas, motion sickness, and other digestive issues. Mix the ingredients and rub over the stomach, or add 1 or 2 teaspoons to bathwater. To personalize, alter this formula, but do not use "hot" oils, such as peppermint, thyme, and black pepper. Do not use hot oils in the bath, as they can irritate or burn the skin.

Nerve Pain Blend

Ingredients

1 ounce St. John's wort or vegetable oil

4 drops chamomile oil

3 drops helichrysum oil (optional)

3 drops marjoram oil

2 drops lavender oil

Directions

The Nerve Pain Blend will relieve pain when applied regularly. Simply mix the ingredients and apply topically. If available, substitute St. John's wort oil for vegetable oil, as it is more effective in combating nerve pain. Purchase St. John's wort at any natural food store.

Poison Ivy Treatment

Poison Ivy Treatment Oat Bath

Ingredients

4 cups quick-cooking oats

3 drops of any mainstay oil

1 cup Epsom salts

1 drop peppermint oil

A square of double-layered cheesecloth

Directions

If the survival shelter is out in the wilderness, a poison ivy treatment is a must. Put all essential oils and the oats in a cloth bag and place the bag into a lukewarm bath. Soak in this bath several times a day. As an alternative to a bath, sponge it on after mixing the essential oils with a cup or 2 of oats dissolved in hot water.

Poison Ivy/Oak/Sumac Remedy

Ingredients

3 drops lavender oil

3 drops peppermint oil

3 drops cypress oil

1 tablespoon warm water

1 tablespoon apple cider vinegar

1/2 teaspoon salt

1 ounce calendula tincture

Directions

This tri-remedy will help cure skin irritation from poison ivy, poison oak, and sumac. Simply dissolve the salt in vinegar and water, in a jar or bottle, and mix in the oils and calendula tincture. Save the solution in the jar and use multiple times, but always shake the bottle well before using. Apply topically.

Aromatherapy for Bladder InfectionsBladder

Infection Blend

Ingredients

2 ounces vegetable oil

8 drops juniper berry or cypress oil

6 drops bergamot oil

6 drops tea tree oil

2 drops fennel oil

Directions

This blend will cure bladder infections. Mix the oils and rub over the affected area once daily. For bladder infection prevention, add a tablespoon of the oil to bathwater.

Sitz Bath

Ingredients

5 drops rosemary oil

5 drops lavender oil

Directions

Steam a hot bath with waist-deep water and drip in the essential oils. Relax in the water for 5 - 10 minutes. Once the time is up, drain the tub and fill it with cold water; sit for 1 minute or longer. If planning a survival stash, hardware stores sell large plastic tubs that can substitute as a bath. Do this anywhere from 2 - 5 times every day if possible.

Burn Treatments

Emergency Compress

Ingredients

1-pint water, about 50°F

5 drops lavender oil

Directions

For severe and unexpected burns, mix the lavender oil with water and stir, or shake, to spread the oil. Place burned appendage in the water/oil combo for a few minutes. Soak a soft cloth in water and set the compress on the burn, leaving it there for a few minutes, soak it again and then reapply a few more times.

Sunburn Soother

Ingredients

200 IU vitamin E oil

20 drops lavender oil

1 tablespoon vinegar

4 ounces aloe vera juice

Directions

This remedy soothes sunburns and helps heal the skin. Be sure to use aloe vera juice rather than drugstore gel. Mix ingredients in a spritzer bottle or jar, and shake well to disperse them evenly. Use as needed. Place in a refrigerator, cooling the mixture will provide further relief.

Aromatic Fungal Fighter

Fungal-Fighting Solution

Ingredients

8 drops geranium oil

3 drops thyme oil

2 ounces apple cider vinegar

2 drops myrrh oil (optional)

1 tablespoon tincture of benzoin

12 drops tea tree oil

Directions

This blend will cure fungal infections, including athlete's foot. Mix the ingredients in a jar or bottle and shake well. Save the solution in the jar and use multiple times, but always shake vigorously before using. Use the solution as a wash once or twice a day, or topically apply the solution on the affected area. Drugstores sell tincture of benzoin.

Fungal Fighter Powder

Ingredients

14 drops tea tree or lemon eucalyptus oil

5 drops sage oil

8 drops geranium oil

1 drop peppermint oil

1/4 cup cornstarch

Directions

In a reseal-able plastic bag, slowly mix the cornstarch and essential oils, evenly distributing the oil amongst the starch. Zip the bag shut and toss. Break clumps that develop, and store long-term in the sealed bag, in a ceramic or glass bottle, or jar. Apply the powder 1 or more times a day.

Healing Hives

Healing Hive Body Wash

Instructions

2 cups water (or peppermint tea)

5 drops chamomile or 10 drops lavender oil

3 tablespoons baking soda

2 drops peppermint oil

Directions

This body wash will help treat hives. Mix the ingredients; if substituting tea for water, use 4 teaspoons of peppermint leaves with 2 ½ cups of boiling water, allowing to steep for 15 minutes. Strain the leaves and combine the tea water with the remaining ingredients. With a soft cloth or sponge, apply the body wash to the affected area. The itching will be alleviated. Though chamomile is more effective for this recipe, lavender oil may be substituted.

Hives Healing Paste

Ingredients

1/4 cup of the Hives Skin Wash (see previous recipe)

3 tablespoons bentonite clay (available at natural food stores)

Directions

Mix the ingredients into the Healing Paste. Let sit for 5 minutes or until thick. With a wooden tongue depressor or fingers, apply to the affected area. Allow the paste to dry on the skin for at least 45 minutes. Wash paste off and reapply for an additional 30 minutes if skin is still itchy and irritated.

Totally Tonic Immune Blend

Ingredients

2 ounces vegetable oil

6 drops bergamot oil

6 drops lavender oil

3 drops tea tree oil

3 drops lemon oil

2 drops myrrh oil (expensive, so optional)

Directions

This Totally Tonic Immune Blend will boost the immune system. Mix the ingredients and massage it into body. Though it can be used generically, it might also be used to target specific areas that have a history of physical issues. For instance, if developing a cough or chest cold, massage the ointment into chest. Use 1 teaspoon in a footbath, or 1 - 2 teaspoons in bathwater. Leave out the vegetable oil and this combination can be used in an aromatherapy diffuser, simmering pan of water, or a potpourri cooker. To boost natural immunity, use any of these methods a handful of times a day.

Energy Boost for Fatigue

Ingredients

2 ounces vegetable oil

8 drops lemon oil

2 drops peppermint oil

2 drops eucalyptus oil

1 drop cardamom oil (optional)

1 drop cinnamon leaf oil

Directions

If feeling exhausted from bugging-out, then this Energy Boost is for you. This solution combats fatigue, making the user alert for whatever awaits ahead. Simply mix the ingredients together and add 2 teaspoons to bathwater, 1 teaspoon to a footbath, or massage into skin. Leave out the vegetable oil and this combination can be used in an aromatherapy diffuser, simmering pan of water, or a potpourri cooker – or, for use as an air spray, combine with 2 ounces of water. Though the cardamom oil is optional, we recommend it for use in the massage oil.

Aromatherapy Sore Throat Treatment

Throat Gargle

Ingredients

½ cup warm water

4 drops marjoram oil

½ teaspoon salt

Directions

Sore throats are the worst, and even more so when in a survival situation. To relieve this issue, mix the ingredients and shake to spread the oils and dissolve the salt. Use for throat spray or gargling. For the best results, gargle every half hour until relief ensues. Continue gargling several times a day until fully healed.

Lavender Neck Wrap

Ingredients

2 cups hot water

2 drops lavender oil

1 drop tea tree oil

 2 drops bergamot oil

Directions

For this soothing lavender neck wrap, combine the essential oils with water. While the solution is still warm, soak a flannel cloth in the solution, wring it out, and wrap it around the affected area. For the best results, cover wrap with a towel to keep the heat in. Before it grows cold, remove it from throat. Use the wrap as often each day as necessary.

Toothache Blend

Ingredients

1 teaspoon vegetable oil

1 drop orange oil

4 drops clove bud oil

Directions

To soothe a painful toothache, mix the ingredients and dab a few drops on the affected area. Do this every half hour until the pain recedes. If you or your child do not like the "hot"-ness of the clove oil, replace it with chamomile oil. Though less effective, it will relieve pain. Apply the blend as often as needed.

Toothache Blend

Ingredients

1 tablespoon vegetable oil

3 drops tea tree oil

3 drops lavender oil

Directions

Infections are most often the cause of earaches. The antiseptic Ear Rub Blend will eliminate the infection and stave off further infection. Simply mix the ingredients and rub around the affected ear and along the side of the neck as well. If the patient is a child, halve this dilution (1-2 drops essential oil to 1 tablespoon carrier oil). Apply 2 to 4 times daily, particularly before sleep..

Conclusion

Now that we know all about essential oils – where they originate, how they are extracted, their benefits and properties, and the different methods of administration – we can start to assemble a survival kit.

The various benefits of essential oils and their properties are countless. The mainstay oils should be the primary focus to begin with, as their base pure components cover many maladies and injuries and when blended, can be even more effective in treatments of additional medical issues.

Used as a supplement or as the go-to treatment, the applications of essential oils in medicine have survived for centuries and will likely survive centuries more. When it comes down to it, we do not need to rely on pharmaceuticals; essential oils, herbs, and plenty of other natural ingredients can help treat any number of ailments and injuries.

When the SHTF, access to pharmaceuticals will likely be limited or eliminated altogether. Alternatives to our modern-day standard will equate with survival when no other option exists.

58

References:

http://www.doomandbloom.net/essential-oils-as-medicine/

http://thesurvivalmom.com/10-reasons-to-have-9-therapeutic-grade-essential-oils-in-your-survival-kit/

http://www.inessence.com.au/a-z-physical

http://health.howstuffworks.com/wellness/natural-medicine/aromatherapy.

www.ingramcontent.com/pod-product-compliance
Lightning Source LLC
Chambersburg PA
CBHW060219290526
45789CB00003B/1328